ALKALINE DIET

The Best pH Alkaline Plant-Based Diet for Beginners with Proven Herbal Medicine Recipe Book for a Revitalized You

Emma Aqiyl

Susan Green Aniys

Shelley Aviv MD

Jonathan Brown M.D.

Felicia Young PhD

Redford E. Gordon

Table of Contents

Introduction

The following chapters will discuss all of the many health benefits to maintaining an alkaline diet as well as the keys to unlocking all of your health potentials. We will look at the chemistry behind the pH scale and how it works and behave within our bodies. We will learn all about why an alkaline balanced diet is the best way to keep your body as healthy as possible.

Maintaining a happy and healthy body can be a real challenge, but within the pages of this book, you will find all of the secrets and tips for making an alkaline-based pH balanced diet a major part of your life with high-impact solutions and surefire methods for creating a healthy pH balance in your own body chemistry.

We will also look at some amazing meal ideas to keep you going strong on the alkaline diet all day every day. Don't miss a single meal with these new and exciting meal ideas. Never be in the dark again! After reading this book, you will know everything you need in order to create and maintain a healthy and satisfying alkaline diet.

There are plenty of books on this subject on the market, so thanks again for choosing this one! Every effort was made to ensure it is full of as much useful information as possible. Please enjoy!

PART 1

Chapter 1: What is the Alkaline Diet?

We eat the foods that we eat for all kinds of different reasons. Sure, from an evolutionary standpoint, we eat food so that we can take in calories and convert them into energy in order to fuel our bodies and keep us going throughout the entire day. The food we eat also provides us with the essential nutrients that our bodies need in order to keep them running in an optimal manner.

But we also eat food for pleasure, the sheer joy of tasting something amazing that we truly love. We eat socially. Food has been a way of bringing people together since the very dawn of civilization. Sometimes we use food for comfort and sometimes we use it to mark formal and important occasions. We use food as a proving ground over which to test out new prospective romantic partners.

And yet, for all that food can do for us, so many of us take it for granted and don't seek out ways to make our food work for us. Used correctly, food and nutrition are tools that can turn our bodies into the healthiest and efficient powerhouse that nature intended them to be.

With so many different diets and nutrition plans out there, it can be hard to know which one is right for you. Well, you're reading this book so you already know that you're on the right track!

Indeed, the alkaline diet is a tried and tested way to get the most out of your body. But how does it work? Why does it work? How can eating an alkaline diet optimize your body and health?

The key to understanding the science and chemistry behind how the foods we eat affect us is to understand that just like the fundamental laws of physics, every action has an equal and opposite reaction. Or in other words, everything that we put into our bodies will affect us based on the characteristics of that particular food item. So if we eat a lot of things that cause the same or similar effects on our bodies, we can influence and even control the effects and changes that our body takes by carefully selecting the foods that we eat and what effect they have on our bodies. As the popular saying goes — you are what you eat.

To illustrate, imagine you are walking through the woods and you accidentally brush up against a poison ivy leaf. Well, sorry to say it, but there is a very good chance that you are going to develop an itchy poison ivy rash. If however, you get completely naked and roll around in an entire patch of poison ivy, you are pretty much guaranteed to get poison ivy and a whole lot of it!

Humorous examples aside, it stands to reason that if we know that a particular food or food group has a particular effect on our body, we can effectively control any number of internal body systems by carefully planning and selecting the foods we eat.

So how does the alkaline diet promote health? Well, the alkaline diet is all about balance. So many of the negative health issues in our lives are the result of an imbalance in our bodies. So much of the history of medicine revolves around finding the ideal balances for the human body.

For many, many years, doctors around the world attributed all of our health conditions, whether good or ill, to a balance or imbalance in what they referred to as the "humors". As far back as Ancient Greece and Ancient Rome, there was a near-universal belief that four humors or bodily fluids influenced every aspect of health and temperament, and ill health or ill temperament was the result of deficiencies or excesses on one or more of these four humors. These four humors were black bile, yellow bile, phlegm, and blood. Each of these four humors was associated with a particular personality type and other such characteristics.

When a person came to an ancient doctor with an ailment, the ancient doctor would examine their patient to determine their temperament and along with other factors would determine where their imbalance in humors was, and then they would come up with a treatment plan with the intention of balancing the patient's humors. So in other words, for millennia, the goal of medicine has been to achieve balance in the human body.

And while many of the theories and practices of ancient physicians have long ago fallen out of use in favor of new techniques and schools of thought, modern science has nevertheless confirmed at least some aspects of ancient medicine, namely, the concept of balance itself.

While we don't hear much about black bile, yellow bile, or phlegm anymore in modern medicine, the fourth humor that ancient doctors treated is certainly still extremely prominent in modern medicine — blood.

Blood is still very much our life force just as it was believed by ancient doctors. Blood is the fluid that keeps us living and breathing and a proper medical understanding is absolutely integral to maintain overall good health.

So how can we maintain a good balance in our blood? What aspect of our blood do we even need to balance? What negative effects can we avoid by maintaining balanced blood and what positive ones can we promote?

While those ancient doctors were certainly on the right track, they had a few key factors wrong so, in order to move forward, we are going to need a firmer and more modern grasp of the science behind our health and nutrition.

To understand this concept a little bit better, we need to understand one of the most fundamental aspects of chemistry. This integral part of chemistry and science as a whole is known as the pH balance or the pH scale. We are going to learn all about the pH balance or the pH scale and how it can affect our bodies in a positive way in the following chapters. First, we will learn what a pH balance is.

Chapter 2: What is a pH Balance?

The first thing we need to understand on our journey to the perfect internal balance via the alkaline diet is exactly just what the pH balance is. Furthermore, we need to understand how the chemical characteristics of a substance or fluid play a role in determining where it falls on the pH scale.

What exactly does the pH scale measure? In short, the pH scale is a measure of the acidity or basicity of solution in which the solvent is water. Such a solution is known as an aqueous solution. In other words, when a substance is dissolved in or is otherwise mixed with water, it can then be tested and measured on the pH scale.

An aqueous solution can be defined as either an acid or a base, as this is precisely what the pH scale is meant to determine. An aqueous solution that is basic is referred to as being alkaline. This gives us a pretty good indication of what the alkaline diet is all about. The pH scale itself is a type of scale known as a logarithmic scale. This means that each equidistant quantified measure is an order of magnitude greater than the previous measurement on the scale. The scale ranges from zero to fourteen, with a neutral pH value being in the middle at seven.

Solutions that have a pH value of less the median value of seven are defined as being acidic, while the opposite scenario, in which a solution is measured to have a pH value of higher than seven — that solution is called basic. Water that is pure and unadulterated is pH neutral which is to say that it should prove to have a pH value of seven when tested, as natural dihydrogen oxide, the chemical name for water is neither a base nor an acid. If that is not the case, then the water should be tested for impurities.

While it is possible for an aqueous solution to have a pH value greater than fourteen or less than zero, these would have to be extremely acidic or extremely basic solutions and would not only be decisively deadly to ingest and even extremely dangerous just to touch. Therefore, for practical purposes, official pH values are nearly always represented on a scale between zero and fourteen.

The pH scale is defined by a set of international standards that are determined and agreed upon by an international scientific body. There are several ways to test the pH level of an aqueous solution, with one of the most notable ones being the use of a glass electrode combined with a pH meter. This scientific instrument determines the difference between a pH electrode and a control electrode in terms of their respective electrical potential. This difference in the electrical potential of a solution relates directly to the acidity of the solution and can therefore be used to give it a standard value.

Another very popular and frequently used means by which to test the pH value of an aqueous solution is by using one of the various compounds known as pH indicators.

A pH indicator is generally some kind of substance that when mixed with an aqueous solution results in a chemical reaction that will literally change the color of the solution, and by examining and comparing the color of the resulting solution, the pH value of the solution can be determined. There are other pH indicators that indicate the pH level of a solution by chemical reactions that result in other physical indicators such as odor for example.

However, by far the most common variety of pH indicators are visual in nature, generally based around color.

One of the most common types of pH indicators is the naturally occurring family of chemical compounds called anthocyanin. These compounds naturally change color reflects the pH balance of whatever item the compound is found within. Generally, these compounds are found in colored plant leaves or other plant parts. One of the most common sources of these pH indicating compounds is from the leaves of a red cabbage. The reason for this is because it is quite easy to extract anthocyanin from a red cabbage making it the perfect resource for a homemade pH indicator test for either health or educational purposes.

Anthocyanin can be found in many different plants though, such as the leaves of the aforementioned red cabbage, but also in certain flowers such as the geranium, the poppy, and also rose petals. Berries and stems can also house anthocyanin compounds such as blueberries and blackcurrants as well as rhubarb. In short, most plants or vegetables that have reddish, purplish, or bluish color in all likelihood contain at least a small amount of anthocyanin compound. When used as a pH indicator by mixing it with an aqueous solution, an anthocyanin compound will become redder the more acidic the solution is and will turn from red to purple to blue the more alkaline the solution is.

Another very commonly used pH indicator since medieval times is the substance called litmus which is derived from various species of lichen. In fact, the word litmus itself means colored moss in its original language, Old Norse. Just like anthocyanin compounds, litmus will turn red when exposed to acidic solutions and blue when exposed to basic solutions. You may even be familiar with the term 'litmus test'. It has come to be used very commonly and very broadly as a metaphor for anything that could be used to soundly distinguish between multiple options.

So with pH balance being fundamental to the chemical nature of all kinds of biological material including the foods we eat, how do we know if and how such foods are affecting our health? We will continue learning about pH imbalance in our bodies to find out. The next chapter will go into the science of how pH balance or more specifically imbalance can affect our bodies and our health.

Chapter 3: The Science Behind pH Imbalance

Every single substance in the world has a pH balance and that includes all of us. Sure, we don't make cabbages change color when we pick them up, but our bodies must maintain a certain pH level in order to live and function properly. This pH balance that is naturally maintained in our bodies is called the acid-based balance and it is quite literally exactly what it sounds like — the balance of acidic and basic substances in your body. More specifically though, when we are referring to the acid-base balance of our bodies, we are most often referring to the pH balance of our blood.

The human body is designed with a few systems in place intended to keep the natural pH levels regulated at an appropriate balance between acidity and alkalinity. Both the kidneys as well as the lungs have a very important role to play in this process. As we previously laid out, the pH balance is generally expressed as a value between zero and fourteen, with seven being the neutral value. And remember that pure and unadulterated water should have a pH value of exactly seven. Knowing then that water is neutral seven on the pH scale, and knowing also that our bodies are designed to maintain an even pH balance, it would stand to reason that our blood should have a neutral pH value of seven as well, right?

Well, not quite. And this is a major key to understand the alkaline diet. The ideal blood pH level is not actually a neutral seven but instead generally should be about a 7.40 on the pH scale. This value can vary slightly from person to person, but that is the standard average. And yes, that's right— the human body should have a blood pH level that is a little bit on the alkaline side.

Generally speaking, it is the kidneys and lungs that regulate this pH level, so if they are not functioning normally, the blood pH level can become imbalanced. This kind of pH imbalance can lead to serious medical conditions which are called acidosis or alkalosis depending on which direction the imbalance goes in. It is important to note that these serious medical conditions must be treated by a medical professional and diet alone cannot entirely reverse these conditions.

Now, what we're talking about in this book is the small, minor imbalances that a general practitioner wouldn't be concerned about because they aren't severe enough to have a serious debilitating effect, but that certainly do have your body operating in sub-optimal conditions, and more importantly, the alkaline diet that can have it function far better than you ever imagined possible.

So in order to better understand how the alkaline diet will allow us to correct these small but important pH imbalances, we'll need to have a complete understanding of what could throw our pH out of balance and why it might happen.

As we have established a moment ago, the primary regulators of the body's pH level are the kidneys and the lungs. There are a large number of small systems in our bodies that have their own pH level and regulate them in their own ways, but the two main, body-wide regulators are the lungs and kidneys.

As you are likely already aware, we take in oxygen with our lungs when we inhale and expel carbon dioxide when we exhale. The oxygen that we take in is absorbed inside our lungs and used as fuel by our cells. The waste product that our cells produce by using the oxygen is carbon dioxide. Which is all very simple and pretty straightforward and familiar to all of us but here's the important part — carbon dioxide is slightly acidic. So by making slight adjustments to how much carbon dioxide is released or retained, our lungs are able to make adjustments to the overall acid-base level of our blood.

Similarly, the kidneys being the filtration system for the vascular system have the ability to excrete small amounts of acidic or basic compounds into the blood in order to make slight alterations to our blood chemistry. This is a slow process as compared to the more immediate effect of the lungs' pH regulatory system. So the lungs and the kidneys could be thought of as the short-term and long-term blood pH level regulators of our body.

If the blood pH level is out of balance, then it can lead to one of these two conditions — alkalosis and acidosis. With the standard balanced blood pH level being 7.40, anything below 7.35 is considered acidosis and anything above 7.45 is called alkalosis. Again, it is important to note that these are serious medical conditions and must be treated by a medical professional. It is always best to consult your doctor if you are suffering from these conditions. What we can do, however, is assist our body's natural pH regulation system by maintaining a blood pH level that is within the tolerable limits.

A low blood pH level or in other words, slightly acidic blood is far more common than the inverse and so that it is what we are primarily focusing on — an alkaline diet that will help us maintain a healthy blood pH level.

While any level measured at 7.35 and under is acidosis and needs professional medical treatment, it is far too common for our blood pH level to fall into that 'safe' range of 7.36-7.39 without being at that ideal sweet spot of 7.40. If you want to get the most out of your body, if you want your body to be operating at peak performance, and if you want to live your absolute healthiest life, then the 'safe' level of 7.36 is not tolerable for your body.

If you are truly serious about your health and your wellbeing, then the 'safe' blood pH level of 7.39 isn't even good enough for you. You need to have the absolute optimal blood pH level and you will settle for nothing but a perfect 7.40. Continue on reading in the next chapters and we are going to show you how.

Chapter 4: Why Alkaline is Best

If our body's pH level is all about balance, then why would maintaining an alkaline diet be superior to an acidic one? Shouldn't we be consuming a perfect balance of alkaline and acidic foods and nutrition? If those are among the questions you are now asking yourself, then you are on the right track. Those are great questions to ask.

There are several reasons why an alkaline diet is a crucial component in maintaining a healthy body and blood pH level. Remember that magic number? The ideal pH level for our blood that will allow our body to operate optimally? That is right — it was 7.40. And do you remember what the pH value for perfectly pure, unadulterated water is? That is right — it was a perfect seven. So what that means, of course, is that the ideal blood pH balance is in fact slightly alkaline at 0.4 units more basic than water.

So we can see already that in order to maintain our ideal pH balance, we will need to intake more alkaline foods than acidic foods. Of course, that is not to say that you can never consume anything acidic. In fact, it is important to have acids as well in order to maintain balance. We just need to be perfectly aware that our body does in fact require a slight alkaline balance and so we should be mindful of this when we plan our meals and overall diets.

This balance may also be reflected in the foods we choose to eat. They don't necessarily need to be extremely alkaline in order to transfer to us the health benefits we are looking for. They may only need to have a slight pull on the alkaline side of the scale. It all depends on our individual bodies and what they are in need of. And of course, everything scales. So a lot of a slightly alkaline substance may have the same value as a little of something with a higher alkaline value. Remember as well that the pH scale is logarithmic which is to say that each unit is exponential to the value of the previous unit. That means that consuming something with an alkaline value of nine would be ten times more alkaline than something with the alkaline value of eight. This is why we need to be careful when consuming anything that is alkaline or acidic. Things can become unhealthy or even dangerous in a real hurry. So, remember to plan ahead and do everything in moderation.

Another equally surface-level reason why it is important to consume a healthy amount of alkaline rich foods is because whether we are aware of it or not, many if not most of the foods we eat on a regular basis are either slightly or moderately acidic. Some very common foods and beverages even go as far as being highly acidic.

Now, again, it bears repeating that this does not mean that you cannot or should not consume these types of acidic foods and beverages at all. In fact, some of these acidic foods and beverages are very healthy and high in essential nutrients. The important thing, however, is to be aware of how much acidic substances we are consuming and how acidic those substances are.

Do you like fruit juices? How about coffee? Those are two great examples of highly acidic beverages that many of us consume on a regular basis. That is not necessarily a bad thing but just think about this — are you taking in the necessary amount of alkaline foods or liquids in order to maintain a healthy and optimal balance?

And what's more, it can often be a good deal more complicated than whether the particular food item that we are consuming is acidic or alkaline on a surface level. What makes the important difference is how the item we consume affects our blood pH level after it has been metabolized. And that could, in fact, be a good deal different than what it might seem to be based on the original acidity or alkalinity of the food item in question.

Another very important reason to remember to include alkaline foods in our diet in order to maintain a good acid-base blood balance is that an acid rich environment is considered by medical professionals to be a hotbed of disease and illness. And remember, it doesn't take much to become imbalanced in one's blood levels, so even a minor imbalance could quickly become a breeding ground for all manner of illness and health problems that you will absolutely want to avoid.

Just by remembering to consume a healthy and appropriate amount of alkaline foods and drinks, we can be safeguarding ourselves from any number of serious health concerns that could be lurking in our very blood. If you want to kill all of those potential illnesses dead before they become a real concern, you will need to act now and ensure that you are consuming an appropriate amount of alkaline foods.

This is the very topic that we will be going into next. We now know how important it is to maintain a good acid-base blood balance. We now know what that optimal blood pH balance is. And most importantly, we now know the dangers associated with having blood that is too acidic, and why it is so common for us to have a blood pH level that skews a little bit too acidic but not enough to go into full acidosis.

Equipped with this crucial information, we can now move on to learning about how to apply these factors to our everyday lives. Now, we are going to learn everything we need to know about how to create and maintain a balanced blood pH level, and all the tips and tricks to make it easy and straightforward.

Are you ready to have a body operating at optimal health? Are you ready to get the most out of your diet? Are you ready to prevent disease and illness that you didn't even know you were susceptible to?

Then continue on reading on, because all of your questions are about to be answered.

Chapter 5: Creating an Acid-Alkaline Balance

In this chapter, we are going to take a look at some of the biggest and best ways to gain control of your acid-alkaline blood levels and ensure that you can maintain them at an optimal level. Many of the things that we are going to talk about here are not just about diet. In fact, even the alkaline diet is not just about diet — it is about habits. It is about keeping good habits, maintaining regular health goals, and being in tune with your own body.

There are plenty of signs and symptoms that you may notice in the event that your body is too acidic. It is very likely that you will be experiencing chronic fatigue if your body is too acidic. Even if it seems that though you have been sleeping enough, you may still feel this way. Other symptoms of overly acidic blood are pain, headaches, joint pain, and stiffness.

Generally, people with acidic blood express an overall feeling of sluggishness and lethargy — sometimes even depression. It is also associated with a sense of irritability and a dulling of the mental faculties.

Obviously, if you are experiencing any of these symptoms, it will be in your best interest to correct them to the best of your ability. There are lots of ways to make your blood more alkaline and we will look at a few here.

First of all, you will want to make sure that your symptoms or feelings are in fact coming from a pH imbalance. In order to do that, you will need to check your blood pH levels regularly in order to maintain an up-to-date record of your pH levels. You can do this very easily with simple, inexpensive home testing kits available online and at many drug stores. You can get an instant and highly accurate reading and find out exactly where your body's pH balance is sitting. These simple test kits can help you make healthy and informed decisions about your personal health based on accurate and current information. This is a great, convenient, and inexpensive way to always be on top of your health.

Now, before we get into specific diet plans, let us talk about some changes that we can make to our diet in a general sense that will help improve our blood pH levels. One such thing that we can do to ensure that we are maintaining appropriate levels of acidity in our blood is by making sure that we eat more greens and dark-colored vegetables in general. Greens are not always the most popular foods to eat despite their great reputation and association with good health. But there are ways to make greens and other veggies fun and exciting and taste great.

You could try new recipes and try new types of veggies that you have never tried before. If you already love veggies, try to make sure that you get a good amount on a regular basis, if not every day. Even if you have a particular proclivity for veggies, it's easy to leave them out on occasion. Try to avoid that tendency.

And if you don't like veggies, maybe it has something to do with a reduction in their appeal on account of processed foods and excessive artificial sugars. Simply by cutting these things out of our diets as much as possible can dramatically reduce cravings for said items and make good, nutrient-rich foods like dark, green veggies far more appealing.

Either way, try to experiment with new ways of getting your veggies and making them fun and enjoyable. Try keeping some prepared in advance so that you always have a quick and healthy snack.

Here is another quick tip for general health and well-being. Every morning, the first thing you do when you wake up should be to drink a great big glass of ice-cold water as fast as you can. Why? Well, it's quick and it's easy, it costs nothing, and it has all kinds of great health and wellness benefits both short-term and long-term. First of all, the most immediate benefit is that ice-cold blast of invigorating water will snap you wide awake quicker and more effectively than any caffeinated beverage.

What's more, there's nothing better than an icy surprise to jump-start your body and kick your metabolism into a high-gear first thing in the morning. And because our friend water is completely calorie-free, that basically amounts to an energy boost and metabolism enhancer for free, metabolically speaking.

And do you want to take this brilliant life hack one step further and bring it into our alkaline friendly lifestyle? Add just a touch of lemon to that morning burst of water, or better yet, all the water you drink and you will get all the previous benefits plus that boost to your body's alkalinity that you need to function at peak efficiency. This may seem counter-intuitive given that lemon is acidic, but remember, it is not always about the acid-alkaline balance of the compound itself. It is how our bodies metabolize that compound. And lemon, being a well-known metabolism booster, will give you that alkaline push you need.

Of course, sometimes it is about the actual acidity of the food we are eating. Specifically, it is about the amount of acidic foods we are eating. If you find that you are suffering from symptoms of acid reflux, kidney stones, low bone density, or anything else associated with high body acidity levels —

that is almost certainly a strong indication that you should be strictly limiting your intake of acidic foods.

This goes of course for any of the obvious culprits like tomato sauce or spicy foods, but there are some less obvious foods that metabolize into an acidic by-product in our bodies that we should be cautious of as well. This includes many processed cakes and cereals, often grain such as rice, oats or pasta, and even certain nuts like peanuts or walnuts. The key here is to just always be aware of what we are consuming and keep everything in moderation.

Beverages as well should be kept in moderation especially coffee and alcohol since both of which are associated with many negative health effects when consumed in excess, far beyond body acid-alkaline balance.

Chapter 6: Alkaline Diet for Vegetarians

Don't let the title fool you, this isn't just for vegetarians. The alkaline diet is great for anyone and everyone. If you are already a vegetarian — great, you are already in a great spot to maintain an amazing alkaline diet. If you're not a vegetarian, that's okay too. Remember in the previous chapter when we said that it is not necessarily about how acidic the foods we eat are but the quantities? Well, that goes for meat. Most meats are extremely acid forming in our bodies.

That means that while they may not be acidic to the taste or even particularly acidic on a pH test, they metabolize in our bodies into an acidic by-product. So naturally, most alkaline diet meal plans are going to be either vegan or vegetarian, or just very light on the meat and dairy. That doesn't mean, of course, that you need to completely remove meat from your diet, but if you choose to continue eating meat, you will need to be highly aware of the quality and quantity of the meat you consume. Keep it moderate and make sure to maintain good health otherwise and you should be okay.

But speaking of acid-forming diets, what so bad about them? We have seen some of the symptoms of having a seriously acidic blood pH level, but what if we're just prone to eating a little bit on the acid-forming side? Well, simply by virtue of the fact that we live in a modern world with modern luxuries and modern conveniences, most of our diets have strayed away from a good, healthy acid-alkaline blood balance, and maybe some of us without even knowing it is may be living with a chronic condition that results from such a diet known as 'chronic low-grade metabolic acidosis'.

This is what happens when our diet leans to the slightly acidic side for an extended, if not an indefinite amount of time. And the reality is that unless we take active steps to counteract this condition, it is highly likely that we will all succumb to it eventually, if not already. That is just the nature of the world we live in and the habits and practices of the industries and populations of our societies.

So if you are suffering from a form of low-grade chronic metabolic acidosis, perhaps without even knowing it, what are the signs? For one thing, you may notice some weight gain. This is a result of inefficient metabolic function on account of long-term low-grade acidosis. You may also suffer from pronounced but unspecific aches and pains. These will often be in the joints or even the bones. This type of pain associated with low-grade acidosis is likely the result of an acid buildup in the joints and bones.

Acid reflux, predictably, is also a good sign of this prevalent condition. But that is not the only part of your digestive system that can be affected. Long-term, low-grade acidosis can also cause a number of other digestive issues like intestinal cramping, irritable bowel, and generally poor digestion.

A whole host of other issues could manifest if you are one of the high percentages of people who unknowingly live day to day with a chronic case of low-level metabolic acidosis. Chronic fatigue and a general feeling of tiredness and muscle weakness may result. As can a number of other issues like skin problems, bone loss, kidney stones, receding gums, and urinary tract problems. So if you find that you have three or more of the many possible symptoms, then at least eighty percent of your caloric intake should be from alkaline-forming foods. The remaining twenty percent can more or less be of your choosing, but you may find high protein food items to be helpful.

A nice, quick and easy way to boost your body's alkalinity is by drinking beverages that are alkalizing. Spring water is one such naturally occurring source of alkalizing water. Also, water with a dash of lemon juice just as mentioned earlier. Green tea or ginger root tea will also have a similarly alkalizing effect.

You'll want to make sure that you are focusing primarily on eating whole foods. So that means vegetables and fruits, as well as root crops like potatoes and turnips. Also nuts and seeds can be an excellent alkalizing source and also a very strong source of protein. Beans are generally a good choice as well, although lentils, in particular, are renowned for their excellent alkalize boost. And when consuming grains, just remember that it is always best to consume whole grains.

Whether you are pursuing an alkaline diet to target a specific issue, or if you just want to have the healthiest body you possibly can, you are going to want to eliminate as much processed and artificial foods as possible. In fact, that goes for everyone, no matter what. Processed and artificial foods are doing anybody any favors, but they will certainly cause your body's blood pH level to lean to the acidic side. Refined sugars and added sugars rank very high up on the list of these types of foods that should be avoided at all cost. And refined white flour isn't doing you any favors either. In fact, some say it can be just as bad as refined sugars.

And while we are on the topic of eliminating things, if you can handle giving up coffee or any other caffeinated beverages, you will be giving yourself a major advantage on the path to a balanced blood pH level.

There are certain foods and nutritional elements that are acid-forming but that our bodies still need to function properly. These are things that we will have to keep a particularly close eye on in order to monitor amounts of intake. This includes essential fats, as well as pasta and other grains. If you are choosing to continue eating meat, then it should also be noted that meat and fish should both be consumed very sparingly and should also be very closely monitored and limited.

Finally, when it comes to dressing up your greens, namely when being consumed as a salad or being cooked, make sure to use high-grade and healthy fats like extra-virgin, cold-pressed olive oil, avocado oil, and coconut oil. All of which bring along tons of health boosts and benefits in addition to their alkaline-forming properties.

Chapter 7: Alkaline Meal Ideas

Now that we are fully informed and equipped to make good nutrition choices in regards to acid-alkaline blood balance, it is now time to put together some meal plans so we can put all of what we have learned into practice. We are going to look at a prime example of everything you might eat in a day to get the most out of your body.

This particular example isn't about limiting calories of eliminating any particular foods or food groups, so if you have any particular calorie counts you need to stay within, or if you are eliminating certain food groups from your diet such as meat or dairy, you may have to adjust accordingly. Just make sure that if you're replacing anything, to replace it with something of a similar acid-alkaline value, and that it serves that same food role as the replaced item. That is to say, replace proteins with proteins, carbs with carbs, et cetera.

And if you are not calorie counting, obviously use your best judgment here but there is no limit to how many alkalizing foods in the fruits and vegetable categories you can eat. Certainly, you should be limiting acidic foods like meats, dairies, grains, and processed foods if for no reason than to keep your acidity levels down, but fruits and vegetables especially the ones that are particularly alkalizing, you can eat to your heart's content.

So with that said, let's take a look at what our alkaline diet morning might look like.

We wake up nice and early in the morning, refreshed and ready to tackle our day because our healthy, alkaline-rich diet is allowing us to get the sleep we need and preventing our bodies from feeling overly fatigued. The first thing we do is get an ice-cold glass of water, squeeze some fresh lemon juice into it and drink the whole thing as fast as we can. As fast as we can without getting a brain freeze that is!

So now we're going to want to have a nice satisfying breakfast. Today, we are going to do a veggie scramble. Sounds great, doesn't it? This breakfast is going to consist of one or two eggs that we are going to scramble up with green onions, spinach or bok choy or any other leafy greens, and then some chopped bell peppers and diced tomatoes. You can even try it as an omelet if you like. Or even an egg-white omelet if you're feeling really healthy.

Or better yet, if you really want to go healthy, why not try that same breakfast, but as a tofu scramble instead of scrambled eggs. It's easy and delicious. Just replace the eggs with a handful of diced, firm tofu. You can season your tofu however you like, but we recommend trying a chili-style seasoning for some nice, tex-mex style breakfast burritos. Wrap optional.

After that amazing breakfast, we're going to have a nice productive and active morning. If we feel the need for a snack before lunch, we'll have maybe a fruit like an apple or a pear, maybe a banana or a handful of nuts or seeds. An ideal choice would be pumpkin seeds or almonds.

If you're anything like us, that already sounds like an amazing and healthy, nutritious day, but we haven't even gotten to lunch yet. So what might we enjoy for our midday meal on this ideal alkaline diet day? Why limit ourselves, let's look at a couple of options.

For one, we could try some lentil soup. This packs a nice alkalizing punch as it is but combine that with some steamed green like broccoli, carrots, onions, or kale, and you've got a powerful meal. Heck, why not steam up a mix of all of those veggies. Try a light olive oil-based salad dressing on the steamed veggies for some extra flavor.

As delicious as that sounds though, we still have another option. If you're still of the animal eating persuasion, you could try a nice big salmon steak, still a far healthier choice that its terrestrial cousin, served with some mixed greens which could include cucumber, carrots, tomatoes, and broccoli, among pretty much any other fresh veggies you would like. Similarly, you can season that with a light vinaigrette of your choice, but we particularly recommend a lemon and dill based one.

After all that amazing nutrition, you must be ready for a snack! Fight off that mid-afternoon slump with a nice alkalizing snack. This one you can keep nice and simple. Try a simple hard-boiled egg, seasoned with sea salt and fresh ground pepper to taste and a garnish of your choice if you're feeling fancy. Or if you're not inclined toward the animal-based foods, try a straightforward but delicious snack consisting of strips of sweet bell peppers, celery, or carrots, or a mix of all is always an option!

Finally, it's time for dinner and this is where you remaining meat eaters are going to have your way. You can have up to four ounces of your favorite meat, whatever that might be, but we highly recommend that if you must have meat, try to stick to something along the lines of fish, chicken, or other types of light poultry. You can serve this with a side of yam or sweet potatoes, baked or prepared in your favorite way and a nice simple garden salad with mixed greens and a light dressing of your choice.

Or for the plant-based folks, you can indulge in some pasta, but try to find or make pasta made from rice or quinoa, or other grains than wheat. Then you can top your pasta with all kinds of delicious veggies like broccoli, zucchini, and garlic. And then garnish with some olive oil and salt and pepper. Now you've had yourself a fresh and healthy food day!

PART 2

Acid reflux is one of the most common ailments affecting adults today. This is due to the notion that there are so many contributing factors and catalysts that can spawn its symptoms. As a result, educating oneself on the best ways to care for the symptoms of reflux is paramount for avoiding and overcoming them once they arise.

Evidently, a common refrain for most reflux sufferers is to avoid foods and drinks that are spicy and or fizzy. While these are certainly helpful approaches to take, you are well advised to consider approaches such as increased exercise for maintenance of overall health, avoiding certain exercises altogether if you are already suffering from severe GERD, implementing dietary changes such as limiting coffee intake, cutting back on peppermint and avoiding highly acidic foods.

But acid reflux symptoms are not caused solely by poor dietary choices alone. Indeed, smoking in excess and excess alcohol consumption are also consistent contributing factors that can induce acid reflux symptoms leading to GERD and Barrett's disease. Leveraging the knowledge presented in this book with regard to the specific dietary and lifestyle changes you must implement, along with acquiring a deeper understanding of the particular scientific reasons for acid reflux, will allow for an informed perspective so that your approach to the symptoms presented is equipped with the most up-to-date and effectual information.

When equipped with these strategies and general knowledge concerning acid reflux, you will certainly be at a distinct advantage when you are confronted by the painstaking and, at its most extreme, life-threatening, symptoms of acid reflux.

Chapter 1: Chronic Acid Reflux & Its Serious health Implications

Acid reflux is the result of abundant backflow of acid for your stomach into the esophagus. Anatomically, when your lower esophageal sphincter (LES) becomes weakened by, among many causal factors, continually consuming a high diet, acid can flow back into your esophagus causing acid reflux. Consequently, there are numerous symptoms that are spawned by acid reflux including, most notoriously, heartburn and indigestion. While high acidity in the gut is common for everybody and is often devoid of serious health concerns if occurring on a minimal basis, serious health concerns can develop if high acidity can persist for a prolonged period of time. If left unattended and without measures of control put in place, in many instances, these health issues will lead to hospitalization or even death. In the most serious cases, chronic long-term heartburn, known as Gastroesophageal Reflux Disease (GERD), Barett's esophagus and esophageal problems can arise due to uncontrolled and unaddressed chronic acidity. Some of these most serious ailments are the remnants of years of neglecting the symptoms of acid reflux, particularly after big meals. Over time, the backflow of acid from your stomach damages your esophagus causing erosion of the layers lining the walls of the organ. This inflammation often leads to very painful swelling in esophagus called esophagitis and is accompanied by a painful swallowing feeling. In addition, esophageal ulcers are the most common ailment of an inflamed esophagus. In fact, GERD is the main cause of these ulcers in the lining of the esophagus. Moreover, painful swallowing, nausea, chest pain contribute to a lack of sleep which perpetuates many of these symptoms simplify virtue of that fact that your body is not getting the required rest to overcome these symptoms. As soon as these symptoms arise, be sure to consult a doctor too so that you can be prescribed medication to treat the symptoms before they grow into more serious, persistent conditions. Acquiring medial intervention is especially important when dealing with an ulcer; indeed, ulcers are extremely harmful to the lining of your organ and can be incredibly persistent if left unattended and given time to grow.

Even more, if your highly acidic diet remains the same as before the ulcer, this contributing factor will only enhance the growth of your ulcer and some of your other symptoms. Over time, the scarring of the lining within your esophagus will lead to scar tissue build up, thereby narrowing the esophagus altogether. Swallowing food and drinks will be made much more difficult as a result and may require a surgical procedure to expand the esophagus. These narrow areas of your esophagus are called strictures, and will likely lead to dangerous weight loss and or dehydration. Avoiding a procedure through immediate medical treatment of high acidity is clearly the preferred approach; but once these strictures block your esophageal pathways, a surgical procedure will be required.

Another common ailment of high acidity that affects many people is Barret's esophagus. Specifically, around 10%-15 of people who suffer from GERD will begin to also develop this painful condition, which results in dangerous changes in cells due to excess stomach acid. Thankfully, less than 1% of those who suffer from Barret's esophagus will actually develop esophageal cancer. If intervened early enough in the process, doctors are able to remove any of these abnormally developed cells through a procedure known as an endoscopy, whereby doctors will insert a flexible tube accompanied by a small camera into your esophagus. However, those who have GERD are at a, albeit slightly, increased risk of developing esophageal cancer. Even still, be sure to consult a doctor as soon as your symptoms reach a persistently painful level so that proactive measures and treatment can be implemented to quell your pain, and inhibit the growth of cancer cells.

If there is a long history of esophageal cancer in your family, you will be at an increased risk of developing this cancer as well, especially if you attain medical treatment after a prolonged period of time experiencing symptoms of high acidity.

If you are aware of having a family history of esophageal cancer, make sure to ask your doctor for a regular endoscopy to find and mitigate the growth of improper cells. Moreover, tooth decay is a very common symptom of excess stomach acid as it wears down the outer layer of your teeth (enamel). As a result, this can lead to excess cavities and weakened teeth. In a recent study, researchers found that over 40% of GERD patients showed significant tooth decay, along with 70% of patients whose reflux had managed to reach the upper esophagus), compared to only 10% of those patients that had no symptoms of reflux. Certainly, reading about the symptoms that accompany stomach acid is disconcerting and worrisome. Nonetheless, being aware of the symptoms and knowing the early signs of their emergence will mitigate the risks of cancer and other chronic ailments like GERD and Barret's esophagus.

So, what can you do about these symptoms and potentially life-altering health concerns if you are experiencing excess stomach acid? Initially, and rather obviously, begin by assessing your diet. If you typically consume large meals, cut down your portions by at least 25%, and avoid eating right before you sleep. The latter is especially important for your digestive track as your body has to work harder to digest food whilst you are asleep and when your body's organs are supposed to be at rest. Also, limit your chocolate and coffee intake. Typically, medical professionals recommend limiting your coffee intake to only 2-3 cups per day at the most. If these levels are exceeded, your body's acidity levels will climb to healthy proportions and heighten your likelihood of acquiring the aforementioned symptoms. In the same way, excess consumption of alcohol and peppermint carry very harmful side-effects. Not mention, smoking is by far the most dangerous to many of your body's organs, especially the esophagus. Taking steps to cut back and eventually quit smoking is strongly recommended to not only avoid esophageal cancer and weakened tooth enamel, but for a bevy of other health-related reasons not directly associated with stomach acidity. When consulting a doctor to address stomach acid symptoms, you will most likely be prescribed an antacid, H2 blocker or a proton pump inhibitor (PPI); all three are available by prescription as well as over the counter.

Where GERD is concerned, there are other major factors that you should look out for. These symptoms are not specific to a particular body type or even certain foods. First, heartburn is, as mentioned, a clear indicator of GERD and is usually an only an occasional issue that is known to affect over 60 million people at least once or twice a month on average. However, for the 20 million individuals who suffer from heartburn on a chronic level through GERD, seemingly unrelated symptoms can inevitably result in numerous other health complications. You are well advised to consult a doctor if you find that you suffer frequent heartburn (two-three times per week regularly).

When you suffer from GERD, acid, food, as well as digestive juices tend to flow back into your esophagus from the pit of your stomach. Over time, this results in esophagitis, thereby leaving the king of the walls of the esophagus extremely vulnerable to additional harm through scarring, tearing and even deterioration. Additionally, while the primary symptom of GERD is heartburn, there are likely to be other symptoms that are far more difficult to diagnose for doctors and patients alike. Notably, doctors refer to a symptom known as, "silent reflux," which includes voice changes, chronic coughing, major and prolonged throat soreness, along with hoarseness. Patients may have a sustained sensation of having a lump in their throatier having the constant urge for having to clear one's throat. Another common symptom of GERD is the effect that stomach acid has on your breathing. Indeed, GERD, for instance, can heighten the extreme effects of asthma and or pneumonia. Whether or not patients have a history of lung problems personally or with regard to their family lineage, GERD can cause difficulty in breathing and persistent shortness of breath. However, treating this particular symptom is especially tricky; according to several recent studies, GERD medication, like PPIs, have been shown to increase pneumonia by directly contributing to the growth of harmful bacteria. Also, researchers have found that many prescribed PPIs suppress coughing that is needed to clear the lungs. As a result, your doctor may be forced to consider the function of your lungs when prescribing PPIs when in the process of treating symptoms associated with acid reflux.

Many people with ulcers from acid reflux tend to spit up blood and or see it in their stool. For a point of clarity, be sure to note that Esophageal ulcers are much different than stomach ulcers as they (stomach) are usually due to bacteria. Blood from esophageal ulcers, however, tend to be red or a darker purple-red color. If you find yourself having such symptoms, be sure to contact your doctor immediately. The immediate response from your doctor will likely be a schedules endoscopy mentioned earlier. In addition, you may also be prescribed acid-blocking or acid-reducing meds can treat these dangerous stomach ulcer.

An overarching common symptom of acid reflux is a lower quality of life. According to a 2004 study from Europe, whereby 6,000 GERD patients reported that their quality of life had been significantly diminished due to problems that are associated with drink, food and sleep, along with social and physical limitations. Not to mention, there can be major financial implications from having to buy an abundant amount of medications to treat the myriad symptoms of acid reflux, as well as the possible surgical procedures and endoscopy sessions that may be needed if the symptoms escalate to advanced stages. Moreover, the quality of life for patients of GERD was strikingly similar to heart-attack patients and was even lower, in certain cases, for those patients struggling with diabetes and cancer.

Generally, the healing time-frame for GERD is around 2 to 8 weeks. If allowed to persist without medicinal intervention, symptoms of GERD can inflict a considerable amount of damage. For example, reflux esophagitis (RO) can create visible and painful cracks and breaks in the esophageal mucosa. In order to fully and effectively heal RO, acid suppression for a prolonged period (roughly 3-9 weeks) is required and will likely be the timeframe advised by your doctor. Keep in mind that healing rates will rapidly improve as acid suppression increases.

Chronic stress is also a significant factor in the development, growth and. persistence of acid reflux. Our digestive system, moreover, is intricately associated with our nervous system. When stress presents itself, especially in an overwhelming or uncontrollable manner, our digestive system will then receive a lower amount of blood flow, thus causing various issues. Further, our gut bacteria are implicated in our management of stress at increasing levels, so probiotics are helpful in helping the management of this development.

Chapter 2: The role of Fibre, Prebiotics and Probiotics

Incorporating key changes into your diet can carry massive benefits with regard to dealing with the many symptoms of acid reflux. Specifically, consuming more fiber is an excellent way to mitigate the harsh symptoms. An important point of clarity is the distinction between dietary fiber, defined as edible but non-digestible carbohydrate-based material, and insoluble fiber. Dietary fiber is mainly available in abundance naturally in many cereals, grains, plants, and vegetables as these all play a major role in gastrointestinal health. Given the importance of fiber, and its positive impact in easing the symptoms of acid reflux, many people on average are dangerously deficient in fiber. This deficiency includes both the soluble and insoluble forms of fiber. The main difference between these two forms of fiber are found in their role in digestion; insoluble fiber expedites the travel of foods through the gastrointestinal tract, while solute fibers have been shown to slow the digestion process.

While the varied and, at times, monotonous science concerning acid reflux is still in progress and remains to be settled. Nevertheless, the theoretical benefits of adequate intake of fiber include avoiding trigger foods altogether, as well as the stomach-filling "full" effect of fiber and fewer relaxation reactions of the anti-reflux valve residing between the stomach and the esophagus. Even still, there exists a persistent relationship between acid reflux trigger and the role of fiber. To elaborate, soluble fiber has been shown to induce the body to draw fluid out of already digested food, which then contributes added bulk to your meals which leaves you with a feeling of being "full" for a far more prolonged period of time. As it is commonly found within such sources as barley, peas as well as oat bran, soluble fiber does play an active role in regulating glucose levels and may even contribute to signaling the brain that the stomach is in fact full both during and after eating a meal of any size. Moreover, smaller meals can help acid reflux by refraining from overfilling your stomach. Whereas, insoluble fiber as found within vegetables and whole grains can speed up the passage of stomach contents to your intestinal tract, thereby decreasing your body's propensity for reflux. Additionally, fatty, fried foods are typically much lower in fiber and are also frequently accompanied by the triggering symptoms of regurgitation, indigestion, and heartburn. Indeed, a fiber-rich diet like fresh fruits, vegetables, and whole-grain bread can tend to contribute to fewer instances of reflux symptoms arising. Some dietary fibers are also widely considered to be probiotics. Note the key distinction between prebiotics and probiotics: the latter refers to the specific helpful bacteria itself, with prebiotic referring to bacterial nutrients. In other words, prebiotics are nutrients which are left for bacteria to digest, or, more plainly, fuel to encourage the balanced bacterial growth within digestive organs. Here, the role of fiber in greatly improving the many symptoms of acid reflux is illuminated; this role is as a bacterial intermediary. On the whole, nonetheless, particular items in your diet tend to perform a seemingly minor role in the symptoms associated with acid reflux. Those who suffer from chronic acid reflux are strongly advised to avoid those specific foods that can aggravate painful heartburn and regurgitation; however, eliminating a broad range of food from your diet is no recommenced as it can detrimental to your overall health. Instead, you should note foods and beverages that can trigger acid reflux specifically and root them out from your diet as soon as possible.

There is a tremendous amount of evidence in favor of incorporating a fiber-rich diet into your daily routine. Notably, the benefits are particular to the overall maintenance of your gut and with regard to managing the amount of harmful bacteria native to that region of your body. A study from 2004 that involved over 65,000 people revealed that fiber intake was associated with the improved perception of acid reflux symptoms. Also, this study revealed people who consumed high fiber bread were nearly three times as likely to experience relief of acid reflux symptoms compared to people who consumed bread with lower fiber content. Granted, the reasons for these results remains unknown; however, the authors of the broad study have speculated that the digestive process of fiber can also be a catalyst for enhanced muscle relaxation from the stomach through the esophagus as it tightens the anti-reflux valve.

So, what are the disadvantages of fiber in acid reflux? It is true that fiber is especially helpful when serving to ease acid reflux symptoms, excess fiber consumption has been shown to aggravate the symptoms. A study published in a medical journalism 2014 indicated that consuming a minimum of 10 grams of highly fermentable starches each day can significantly contribute to painful episodes of acid reflux symptoms. An additional study noted that nine participants who were diagnosed with GERD, those patients who consumed a prebiotic known as fructooligo also had elevated instances of acid reflux symptoms than those patients who were given a placebo.

There are many aspects to consider when striving to efficiently manage acid reflux symptoms. Among them, dietary fiber is perhaps the most important or, at the very least, the most consequential. For instance, while being excessively overweight is certainly risk factor as far as GERD is concerned, adequate consumption of healthy fiber will aid in keeping the weight at a healthy level. Excess fiber, however, causes stomach distension in may people, along with enhanced stomach pressure as well as prolonged emptying on the stomach in many cases, all of which have shown to lead to accentuated acid reflux symptoms. Medical professionals specializing in gastroenterology strongly recommend implementing lifestyle changes such as eating smaller sized meals on a frequent basis (as opposed to larger meals a few times per day), limiting overall consumption of carbonated beverages and foods high in salt content with the intent of improving the acid reflux symptoms. Note that women over the age of 50 should try to consume 25 grams per day; on the other hand, men under 50 are strongly advised to consume 38 grams of fiber each day. While consuming more laxatives is often the approach undertaken by people dealing with symptoms of acid reflux, medical professionals advise increasing your fiber content within your diet for maximized results, as well as maintaining your overall health as laxatives can take a substantial toll on your body and its digestive tract. Consuming a higher amount of fiber will strengthen your stool, keep wastes traveling more smoothly through your intestinal tract, along with preventing constipation. During this process of consuming more fibre, be sure to also ensure that you are consuming plenty of water as well; for fiber to have its absolute best effect, it is imperative that your body remain as hydrated as possible to make sure that waste moves smoothly along your intestinal tract rather than building up due to rigidity.

A good source of probiotics and fiber is yogurt, which carries "good" bacteria helpful for overall maintenance of gut health. A healthy gut is paramount for an efficient and well-functioning intestinal tract and digestive system. Prebiotics and probiotics are, essentially, analogous to food for the bacteria in your stomach; bananas, corn, and whole wheat are additional food sources that are high in prebiotics. Moreover, one of the most beneficial aspects of a fiber-rich diet is the notion that high-fiber foods help control your cravings for snacks. Certainly, high fiber diets can help you lose weight as it displaces other calories for overall maintenance of health.

Guarding against illness, fiber-rich diets will also lower your chances of developing major gut-related illnesses such as diverticulitis. This condition, pockets in the walls of colon trap waste as opposed to moving it along. While doctors remain unsure of the direct catalyst(s) for the illness, consuming a high-fiber diet moves waste fervently along through your system. Along with diverticulitis, a high-fiber diet also eases and prevents irritable bowel syndrome— which has also been linked to acid reflux, albeit a rarer, more extreme symptom. Nevertheless, the most common symptom of acid reflux— heartburn— is quelled by a fiber-rich diet.

Probiotics are becoming increasingly linked to the management of the symptoms associated with acid reflux and alleviating these issues. For a more technical explanation, as we are already aware that probiotics are an effective way of balancing the gut bacteria inside of our bodies, they also help combat against a bacterial infection knows as, H. pylori. This bacterial infection usually originates in childhood. This bacteria, found in the stomach, can alter the environment around them through reducing the acidity levels so that they can survive for longer periods of time. By penetrating the lining of the stomach, thereby remaining hidden and protected by the mucous membrane so that the body's immune defenses cannot reach them. In addition, these bacteria tend to secrete an enzyme called urease, which converts urea to ammonia. The presence of ammonia in this instance is significant because it reduces the stomach acidity around the specific area where the bacteria is found. Coincidentally, it is this lower stomach acid that is often mistaken— by doctors and patients alike— for acid reflux. Can probiotics help combat H. pylori? Well, many medical researchers believe that probiotics can, in fact, help battle this bacteria in several key ways. For one, probiotics are believed to strengthen the protective barrier against H. pylori by producing antimicrobial substances, along with competing against H. pylori for what is known as adhesion receptors (space on the lining of the stomach). Also, it is believed that probiotics assist in stabilizing the gut's mucosal barrier. Many researchers even argue that the production of relatively large amounts of lactate is another inhibitory factor of H. pylori due to the possibility that it could lower the H. pylori urease. Not to mention, probiotics may also be effective in modifying inflammation levels by interacting with the epithelial cells that are responsible for managing the secretion of inflammatory proteins in the gut.

Depending on the particular cause of your acid reflux, probiotics can be incredibly useful for alleviating the painful symptoms. Probiotics can be taken in conjunction with an antacid without worry of the antacid overtaking the positive benefits of the probiotic. More importantly, your approach should be to uncover the root of your acid reflux and adjust medical intervention accordingly. Of course, you doctor plays a huge role in this process, especially in diagnosing the specific cause of your acid reflux; still, it is your responsibility to seek medical expertise so that you can tackle the root of the symptoms as opposed to addressing the individual symptoms as they arise. Being aware of the triggers in both the food and drinks that you consume, managing your stress levels regardless of how often they fluctuate, and finding the specific levels of acid within your stomach are critical steps to address the symptoms of acid reflux. More likely than not, the best method of dealing with your symptoms will be to implement a diverse approach that incorporates a range of approaches rather than relying solely on medical intervention.

Chapter 3: Understanding the role of proteins, carbs, AND fats in healing acid damage

In recent years, there have been increasing reports concerning the benefits of a low-carb diet in healing the damage induced by acid damage. This may seem counterintuitive given the notion that the standard treatment for GERD includes the *removal* of certain foods that increase acidity in the stomach, for example, tomato sauces which are believed to be contributing causes of excess stomach acidity. Also, as mentioned in chapter 1, the removal of coffee, alcohol, smoking, and peppermint are other dietary and lifestyle changes that ease GERD symptoms. Additionally, researchers have found that diets with a higher amount of carbohydrates can significantly elevate symptoms of acid reflux. Whereas, a low-carb diet has also been shown to reduce symptoms of GERD. While many health researchers and medical experts have expressed concern over the exceptionally low proportion of daily calories from fat and protein in low-carb diets, as wells calorie levels being considerably lower in these diet than recommended. Nevertheless, the effects of gastroesophageal reflux disease have been shown to be significantly reduced after implementation of a low-carb diet. For a case in point, following a 2001 research study in which 5 individuals with diverse ranges of GERD symptoms and across the age spectrum, engaged in a low-carb diet, each of the 5 research participants showed significant relief of symptoms. Granted, throughout the duration of the study, which spanned 8 months, 3 of the 5 research participants also reduced their coffee intake concurrently.

The concurrent reduction of coffee, coupled with lower intake of carbohydrates, was shown to be effective in reducing symptoms such as heartburn and stomach pain. Interestingly, while coffee reduction was a contributing factor, observations from a few of the participants revealed that exacerbating foods such as coffee and fat are less pertinent when a low-carb diet is strictly followed. In other words, when implementing a low-carb diet, the effects of classic factors like coffee and fat intake are vastly diminished even if their consumption is not significantly reduced. So, whether or not you choose to reduce coffee and fat intake significantly, you are likely to reduce most GERD symptoms by solely undertaking a low-carb diet. Therefore, the logical conclusion to draw from these findings is that a low-carb diet is a significant factor for reducing the symptoms of acid reflux. This conclusion gains even more credibility when considering the propensity for high-carb diets to aggravate GERD symptoms.

In addition to lower carbohydrates, lean sources of protein and healthy fats are beneficial for reducing symptoms associated with acid reflux. Lean proteins found in eggs are a great addition to your diet for reducing acid reflux symptoms; however, they are a problem for many people due to elevated cholesterol. If eggs are an issue for you, be sure to consume only egg whites and refrain for consuming higher fat yolks—which have been shown to elevate GERD symptoms. Moreover, as high-fat meals and fried food typically descries LES pressure thereby delaying emptying of the stomach and boosting the risk of acid reflux, it is in your best interest to choose lean grilled meats, as well as poached, baked or broiled meats. Boosting proteins, in the way, will also provide benefits for your overall health as well. Also, complex carbohydrates, as found in rice, whole grain bread, couscous and oatmeal carry excellent benefits for reducing GERD symptoms and easing any scarring that may already be present in the walls of your esophagus. Specifically, brown rice and whole grains add valuable fiber your diet. Root vegetables such as potatoes are excellent sources of healthy carbohydrates and easily digestible fiber. Remember to refrain from incorporating too much garlic and onion while preparing your meals, which are can commonly irritate the esophagus and stomach lining.

Along with proteins and complex carbs, incorporating healthy fats has great benefits for easing GERD symptoms and other symptoms accompanying acid reflux. A type of nutrient, fat is high in calories but certainly a necessary component of your diet. Keep in mind, however, fats can vary and they do not all have the same effect on your body. On the whole, you are well advised to avoid consuming a high amount of saturated fats as typically found in dairy and meat, along with trans fats found in processed foods, shortening and margarine. As a replacement, unsaturated fats from fish and or plants are recommended; some examples of monounsaturated fats include sesame, olive, canola, sunflower, peanuts, seeds and nuts, as well as butter. In addition, examples of polyunsaturated fats include such oils as safflower, corn, flaxseed and walnut, fatty fish such as salmon and trout, along with soybean.

Some other helpful tips for reducing acid reflux symptoms include chewing gum, as long as it is not spearmint- or peppermint-flavored. Chewing gum increases the amount of saliva production in your mouth and also reduces the amount of acid in your esophagus. While alcohol consumption has already been mentioned in earlier chapters, research suggests that some people begin to experience extreme symptoms after only one drink; if you fall into this category, be sure to experiment with your levels to uncover what amount is best for you. Additionally, during and after each meal, particularly bigger meals, be sure to remain aware of your posture. Generally, it is a good idea to sit up while you are eating and avoid lying flat on your back for at least hours post-meal. Standing up and walking around the room after a big meal can help encourage the flow of gastric juices in the right direction. Further, avoiding eating big meals before bed can help you refrain from overloading your digestive system while you sleep. Digestion increases the overall amount of gastric acid that is present within your stomach. When laying down, LES's ability to inhibit stomach contents from traveling through the esophagus decreases significantly. When operating concurrently, excess stomach acid and remaining in a reclined position for an unexpended period of time create an abundance of acid reflux symptoms. On the whole, consuming a large meal for less than 3 to 4 hours prior to bed is generally not advisable for those suffering from persistent GERD symptoms; however, the timing of these symptoms can certainly vary depending on the individual.

In a 2017 research study on the benefits of healthy dietary changes versus drug intervention, researchers studied the effects of dietary changes to a type of reflux known as laryngopharyngeal reflux or LPR. This reflux is essentially triggered when pepsin, a digestive enzyme from the stomach, reaches the sensitive tissues in the upper section of the digestive tract. Symptoms like throat clearing and hoarseness are common with pepsin in the throat and or upper part of the digestive tract. In the study, the researchers had participants suffering from acid reflux switch to a Mediterranean diet and consuming significantly more water, thereby neutralizing excess acid. In this particular study, participants avoided classic triggers such as coffee, peppermint, alcohol, fatty and spicy foods, chocolate and soda. Another set of participants were given pharmaceutical drugs to ease GERD symptoms.

After a six week timeframe, participants of the study reported a greater percent of declines in their GERD symptoms as those participants that had used drugs to address the symptoms. Granted, the study did not elaborate on the particular ways in which that the diet and increased water consumption eased the symptoms; nonetheless, the Mediterranean diet incorporates eating mostly plant-based fruits and vegetables. In addition, the increased water can mitigate pepsin's acidity levels in the throat. As mentioned, fruits, vegetables and water are great methods of reducing acid reflux and GERD symptoms. With this in mind, the positive benefits experienced by the study's participants is not surprising in the least.

Adjusting your diet for GERD does not require removing all of the foods that you typically enjoy eating. Instead, a few simple changes to your diet if more than enough to address the uncomfortable symptoms of GERD. Your aim in addressing the GERD symptoms should be to create a well-rounded, nutrient-based diet that incorporates a variety of foods that include vegetables, fruits, complex carbs, healthy fats and lean sources of protein. Healing acid reflux damage is made significantly easier when starting with dietary changes that add healthy and diverse foods. Coupled with medical intervention (if required), healthy dietary changes can carry great benefits for healing scarring in your esophagus and stomach, as well as symptoms such as heartburn, bloating and even tooth decay.

Chapter 4: Exercise to reduce acid reflux

When GERD symptoms escalate and you are still in the early stages of implementing dietary changes to address acid reflux symptoms, exercise can be a great option for reducing the symptoms. When GERD symptoms begin to arise, high-impact physical activities like running, skipping rope and jumping exercises. If you are overweight or obese, a weight loss of 10% has been shown to reduce GERD symptoms like heartburn, bloating and reflux. A self-reported analysis study of individuals experiencing GERD symptoms fund that those who reduced their Body Mass Index (BMI) by 2 kilograms or 4.4 pounds or more, along with the circumference of their waist by 5cm or more has improved their GERD symptoms significantly. In contrast, there are also certain exercises that can induce reflux by opening the lower esophageal sphincter (LES) during workouts such as heavy lifting, stomach crunches, or other high impact exercises. When the LES opens, stomach acid travels up into the esophagus causing heartburn. There are some common sense tips concerning exercise for managing GERD symptoms. First, this twice about how much and what you are eating prior to starting your exercise routine. Obviously, less food in your stomach is ideal. If you are too full, you should wait at least 1 to 2 hours before initiating your exercise routine. This will allow for food to pass fro your stomach through to the small intestine. With less food in your stomach while exercising, it is significantly less likely that you will experience the painful and annoying symptoms of acid reflux such as heartburn and bloating. Next, you should choose the food you consume with thought and, in some instances, caution. Generally, you should avoid foods that trigger GERD symptoms (choosing complex carbohydrates is advised). Your stomach does metabolize these foods much faster than others through a process known as gastric emptying. Moreover, diabetics should avoid high fat and high protein foods before exercise due to being more susceptible to experiencing slow gastric emptying. Experts also suggest adjusting your workout if you suffer from frequent GERD symptoms. Starting at a slower pace with workouts that put less strain on your body like controlled walking and controlled weight training in either a sitting or standing position is strongly recommended. Whereas, high impact, high-intensity workouts like running, rowing and cycling and induce acid reflux. Additionally, acrobatic workouts and gymnastics can also disrupt stomach contents. The key is to avoid exercises that jostle the LES and reflux, these are typically positions that put your body in awkward positions like being upside down defying gravity in one way or another.

A great exercise that carries tremendous benefits for improving and relieving acid reflux symptoms and digestion is yoga. One particular study from 2014 found that six months of yoga significantly reduced acid reflux and stomach bloating, along with improved esophagitis. Again, however, try to avoid positions that heighten GERD symptoms. If any of these "lifestyle" changes fail to improve your GERD symptoms during exercise, be sure to consult your doctor about being prescribed medication for acid-suppression. And, of course, engaging in a constant exercise routine is not only very beneficial with regard to improving your GERD symptoms, but also for the maintenance of your overall health.

Chapter 5: How to live a reflux free life?

As you may have already noticed, acid reflex can be induced by an abundance of factors ranging from diet, bad habits, poor sleep hygiene, and many other factors. Clearly, it isn't just as simple as cutting out bad habits and instilling a series of great dietary and lifestyle changes. But whether you are able to successfully implement these changes or not does not, thankfully, hinge on strict adherence to a stringent diet or eliminating some of your favorite guilty habits. But before you can begin to consider stepping into a reflux-free life, you should be cognizant of the stages of reflux and recovery.

Firstly, almost everyone who suffers from GERD begins with normal LES and little to no reflux. The severity level of GERD, therefore, more than likely correlates to best with the overall degree of damage inflicted upon the sphincter. Note, however, that this is not easy to determine. Normally, the amount of damage to your sphincter correlates with the overall severity of acid reflux symptoms. This severity is most often determined by the volume, frequency, and duration of reflux episodes. In turn, these factors will correlate with GERD symptoms such as regurgitation and heartburn. If you are diagnosed with GERD, your strategy for addressing the symptoms and eventually overcoming them should first be to containment. Unfortunately, damage to your LES caused by GERD cannot be reversed by drugs and is permanent. Nonetheless, many patients of GERD have been able to live with these symptoms and with functionality despite damage to the sphincter. Changing simple lifestyle habits, such as sleeping and eating, can significantly decrease and prevent severe reflux episodes in spite of damage to your sphincter.

In Stage 1 of GERD, known as Mild GERD, most adults currently have minimal damage to their LES and tend to experience mild GERD occasionally. Most often, the adults are left with either tolerating occasional heartburn or will have to use over-the-counter acid suppressive medications from the onset of symptoms through its subsequent stages. Typically, when taking drugs to address the symptoms, quality of life for patients is not affected because the medications are very effective in suppressing symptoms. If you choose to take medication to address symptoms, make sure that you are also cleaning up your diet. If you continue to consume trigger foods and beverages, like coffee and certain sauces, for example, the benefits you garner from medication will be minimal and your recovery will be prolonged if not inhibited altogether. Replacing these meals with smaller, leaner meals that do not pose a threat to inducing symptoms of GERD is recommended. This will ease heartburn and lessen the damage to your sphincter.

In stage 2, known as Moderate GERD, symptoms are far more difficult to control and use of prescribed acid-suppressive drugs will be needed. In this stage, reflux is accompanied by symptoms that are far more intense than stage 1. Therefore, medicinal intervention is needed to mitigate the damage and pain caused by these symptoms. Still, many symptoms in this stage can be managed by using acid-suppressive drugs for prolonged periods of time. Keep in mind that over-the-counter medication can provide insufficient relief; whereas, prescription strength medications are needed in order for you to manage GERD symptoms effectively. Additionally, stage 3, or, Severe GERD, can result in a very low quality if life and is generally considered to be an extremely serious problem by medical professionals specializing in GERD. Because prescription grade acid-suppressive drugs and medicinal intervention usually do not control symptoms, regurgitation is frequent. In Stage 3, it is entirely possible that complications associated with erosive GERD are present. Lastly, stage 4, or, reflux-induced esophageal cancer, is quite obviously the most serious stage. The result of numerous years of severe reflux, nearly 16% of all long-term reflux sufferers progress to this extremely advanced stage. Due to the long-term reflux, the esophagus' lining has been heavily damaged, thereby resulting in a high degree of cellular changes. Also, stage 4 is the stage that involves the pre-cancerous condition called Barrett's esophagus and or an even more severe condition called dysplasia. Granted, these conditions are not cancerous. However, they are capable of raising the risk of developing reflux-induced esophageal cancer. Accordingly, at this stage, common GERD symptoms are likely to also be accompanied by a strong burning sensation in the throat, chronic coughing, and persistent hoarseness. A narrowing of the esophagus, or strictures, will also be present in this stage, and can also be characterized by the sensation that food is sticking to your throat. However, this is only a feeling associated with strictures. Notably, this symptom is also caused by esophageal cancer. Keep in mind that stage 4 GERD can only be diagnosed by a medical professional through an endoscopy and from an intrusive biopsy of cells retrieved from the lower esophagus.

A 30-day recovery plan for GERD symptom can be easily broken into weekly steps. In the first week, you will presumably be trying to lean off of the medication that you have been prescribed. A reversion plan of this nature should take into account a variety of approaches that incorporate dietary changes, exercise routines, sleep schedules, and other lifestyle changes. Drinking more tea and water is strongly recommended throughout your 30-day reversion plan, as long as the tea is not peppermint-flavored. Also, in your first week of recovery, be sure to get as much sleep as possible, in conjunction with eating 2 to 3 hours before you sleep. A meal should also be incorporated throughout this entire 30-day stretch. This plan should include egg whites in the morning, instead of coffee switch to tea for your caffeine fix. For lunch, whole grain bread with lean meat- chicken or turkey preferably- with light sauce and a bevy of vegetables. Moreover, dinner should include a balanced meal that provides nutrients and foods that will not induce heartburn. Remember, this meal should be consumed a few hours before bed so that your body has time to properly digest the food. Also, be sure to refrain from lying directly on your back after your meal; as mentioned, this will induce acid reflux symptoms like heartburn and excess bloating.

In week 2, in keeping with the consumption of nutrient-rich food and water consumption from the previous week, you should begin an exercise routine of you have been devoid of routine prior to week 2. A consistent exercise routine will help maintain overall health so that your body has excess strength and energy to overcome the wear and damage inflicted from GERD symptoms. Also, a consistent exercise routine will boost your metabolism so that you can burn off excess unhealthy fats and complex carbohydrates that can cause strain to your body and induce reflux symptoms. In the third week of your 30-day revision plan, you can slightly increase the size of your meals. Still, make sure that the overall size of your meals remain relatively small, with only slight additions where you may see fit. By week three, your exercise routine, water consumption, and sleep habits should be starting to feel more routine and many of reflux your symptoms will begin to diminish. Moreover, leading into week 4, your diet should continue to incorporate nuts, vegetables, fruits, tea, and other plant-based foods and drinks to expedite the healing process. However, the final week of your 30-day recovery plan is vital for sustaining the progress that you have presumably made since the start of the month. It is vital because you must ensure that you do not get too comfortable in your routine that you allow for gradual decline back into the habits that spawned your acid reflux. Pushing through this final week will augment your progress and solidify your path to living a reflux-free life. Specifically, with regard to your diet, you can incorporate the following fruit and vegetable smoothie recipe. Smoothies and healthy shakes are an excellent meal replacement option for optimal health and recovery from acid reflux.

- Add 2 scoops of frozen berries into a 400ml cup
- Add 2 scoops of spinach from a 250ml scoop
- Add 2 tablespoons of Chia Seeds
- Add 2 tablespoons of hemp hearts
- Add 1 tablespoon of peanut butter
- This smoothie should be blended with water to ensure that it is not excessively thick.

CONCLUSION

Good job for making it through to the end of the book. We hope it was informative and able to provide you with all of the tools you need to achieve your goals whatever they may be.

The next step is to put everything that you have learned in this book into practice. Learning more about your body and how it works is always a great place to start and in this book, we learned all about the acid-alkaline balance in our bodies, how the chemistry works, and what are the effects this balance or imbalance can have on our health.

We learned about some of the cutting edge science behind our understanding of pH levels in our body, and how we can fine tune them to the perfect level through our diet and other important practices. The human body is a very complicated and delicate machine, but the more we come to understand it, the better off we are and the more educated we can be in our choices regarding our health and wellbeing.

Given that your acid reflux is likely to exist on a ranging spectrum and will most definitely be different for every individual, this book provides methods of addressing your symptoms and ailments in a manner that is applicable and helpful for whichever stage of the reflux you are experiencing. What's more, the 30-day recovery plan is a great way to ensure that your symptoms are staved off for good once you can utilize medical intervention. If, for instance, you are prescribed drugs to mitigate your symptoms, be sure to use the methods outlined in this book in conjunction with the prescribed amount of medication that your doctor has instructed.

Where your health is concerned, being prepared and informed is critical to seeing that you successfully overcome the ailments that are affecting you.

That is precisely why this book is of value. After reading, you are now informed about the intricate aspects of acid reflux and should feel extremely prepared as you move forward in addressing these symptoms.

Now, it's up to you to take what you have learned in the preceding chapters and apply them into your life. Do you have what it takes to be in full control of your own health and get the very most out of your body? Will you settle for a body that works within tolerable levels, or do you want to maintain peak balance in your life and in your health? Then now is the time to apply all that you have learned and prove it for yourself!

CPSIA information can be obtained
at www.ICGtesting.com
Printed in the USA
LVHW081129310122
709853LV00013B/943

9 781913 710071